Amazing Fitness At 60+

Easy Home Exercises To Gain Balance, Flexibility And Strength.

By

Anna Beckles

CONTENTS

INTRODUCTION

You must get ready if you want to mature gracefully and comfortably.

Our lean muscle mass begins to decline by 1 to 2 percent a year around the age of 50. This muscle loss can significantly decrease our independence while raising our risk of accidents and falls.

What if you were able to regain your strength, equilibrium, and vitality more quickly than you ever imagined? What if you could get significant effects in just 15 days with a tried-and-true training regimen that only requires a few minutes 2 to 3 times a day?

Nearly everyone's daily health, including older adults, benefits from exercise. Seniors should be as active as they can. Exercise can contribute to a longer, healthier life for older adults.

It makes no difference if you're 60 or 100 years old, if your health is excellent or subpar, if you walk kilometers every day or if you have to strain just to get out of a chair.

Amazing Fitness At 60+

will teach you how to change your body and your life, regardless of how fit and healthy you are now.

CHAPTER 1

You Are Not Too Old

Have you stopped working out? Many older adults exercise regularly, but only one in four persons between the ages of 65 and 74 do so. Many people think they are too unfit, ill, exhausted, or simply old to exercise. They're mistaken.

At any age, developing or maintaining a regular fitness program can be difficult; becoming older doesn't make it any simpler. Health issues, aches, pains, or worries about accidents or falls may make you feel demoralized. If you've never worked out, you might not know where to start or feel too old or fragile to meet the goals you set for yourself when you were younger. Or maybe you just think that exercise is boring.

We all understand the benefits of exercise, right? Obviously, we do! But getting started might be very challenging for older individuals. Even if they succeed in starting, many people are unable to maintain a regular fitness regimen due to soreness, sprains, and balance problems. However, exercise is essential for older individuals to live a happy and healthy life!

Age-related physiological changes give rise to a variety of motivations for maintaining fitness. Even though physical fitness offers a wealth of advantages at any age, the health benefits that physically fit seniors experience stand out more. Numerous studies suggest that elders should maintain as much activity as they can without overdoing it. Exercise promotes longer, healthier, and happier life in older persons.

For older folks who are not receptive to the concept or who have never tried anything before, exercising alone can be a little monotonous. Today, there are digital platforms that provide guided classes in addition to Youtube channels run by training professionals that include content specifically created for older folks. The fact that you are not alone is the nicest thing about these platforms. An excellent method to keep regularity and stay on track with your wellness goals is to have a friend who can help you stay on schedule. Humans are social creatures, therefore getting older shouldn't make you lose touch with the outside world, even when exercising.

When starting out on workouts on your own as a senior, it is easy to make mistakes. Take it gently when starting an exercise regimen again. By doing so, you can make sure that your body detects the new motions and modifies itself to react favorably.

As you get older, these may seem like good reasons to take it easy and slow down, but they're actually stronger reasons for getting up and moving. Increased activity can boost your mood, reduce stress, assist you in controlling pain and sickness symptoms, and enhance your general sense of well-being. And intense exercises or frequent excursions to the gym are not necessary to gain the benefits of exercise. Even in little ways, increasing your mobility and activity can have positive effects on your life. It's never too late to get your body moving, improve your health and outlook, and age better, regardless of your age or physical condition.

Everyone is aware of the health benefits of exercise. Did you know that it holds true for people of all ages, including the elderly? You can always get stronger, move more, and take better care of your health.

Including physical activity and exercise in your day can improve your quality of life in a variety of ways. Your balance can be enhanced by regular exercise, which can also increase or preserve your strength and fitness. Additionally, it might lift your spirits and assist you in controlling or lessening the effects of illnesses like diabetes, heart disease, osteoporosis, and melancholy.

Exercise for older persons should focus on endurance, balance, strength, and flexibility, according to experts. Your heart, lungs, and circulatory system will be healthier as a result of brisk walking, dancing, and other endurance exercises. You may find it simpler to climb stairs, mow the grass, and carry out other daily tasks after engaging in these workouts. Lifting weights or using resistance bands are examples of strength training exercises. They can aid with tasks like lifting children or carrying groceries by boosting muscle strength. Falls are a significant health risk for older persons and can be avoided with balance exercises. Exercises that increase flexibility, such as stretching, can help you move more freely, allowing you to bend to tie your shoes or peek over your shoulder as you pull out of the driveway.

Building a balanced exercise plan

Being active is not a precise science. Just bear in mind that combining different physical activities keeps your workouts interesting and helps to improve your health in general. Based on the four foundational elements of fitness, the goal is to identify activities you enjoy. As follows:

1: Balance

This is the kind of exercise that is frequently disregarded. If we do nothing, the systems that control our balance—vision, leg muscles and joints, and the inner ear—break down as we age. As we get older, we all want to be more stable on our feet, which is what balance training does.

For this, tai chi and yoga are excellent, and most gyms and senior centers offer lessons in both. Even DVDs and YouTube videos offer these kinds of workouts. Balance exercises are a part of physical treatment for those who have fallen, and the exercises should continue after the rehabilitation is over. Balance exercises can be found online, and even simple exercises like occasionally standing on one foot might help.

It's better to start keeping balance before an issue arises, but if difficulties start, it's definitely not too late; just seek professional help first.

Why it's beneficial to you: Your posture, balance, and walking style all improve as a result. Your chance of falling or fear of falling is also decreased.

2: Cardiovascular endurance

The ability to perform exercises using your entire body for a lengthy period of time at a moderate to a high level is known as cardiovascular endurance. Your ability to complete daily tasks more easily can be increased by increasing your cardiovascular endurance. Additionally, it can lower your risk of developing conditions including diabetes, heart disease, and stroke.

Why it's beneficial to you: Asthma symptoms can be eliminated, chronic pain can be lessened, blood pressure can be maintained, and heart health can be improved.

3: Strength Training

Regaining the muscular mass we lose as we get older requires an active exercise of the muscles. Strength training enables us to carry out yard work, carry groceries, and lift big objects until old age, which is something we all want to be able to accomplish. Additionally, it prevents the deterioration of our bones, decreases blood sugar, eases joint and back discomfort, and enhances posture.

With workouts like squats and lunges for the legs and bicep curls, flies, and tricep curls for the arms, the goal should be two or three times per week. If you are confused about where to start, you can take a session with a personal trainer or just look up some recommendations online from a reliable source, based on your research on age and ability.

Why it's beneficial for you: Strength training improves balance, builds muscle, and prevents the loss of bone mass, all of which are necessary for maintaining an active lifestyle and preventing falls. For instance, power training can help you cross the street more quickly or prevent falls by teaching you how to respond fast if you start to trip or lose your balance. Maintaining your independence and making daily tasks like opening jars, getting in and out of cars, and lifting objects simpler will be made possible by developing your strength and power.

4:Flexibility

Flexibility is crucial to avoiding muscular cramps, strains, joint pain, and falling as we become older because we naturally lose it as we age. As we age, our muscles become shorter, so we need to stretch them out to improve our range of motion and reduce the likelihood of pain and injuries.

Stretch at least three or four times a week, and warm up beforehand with a steady exercise like arm circles and place marches. After that, hold each stretch for a minute, focusing on the shoulders, back calves, hamstrings, hip flexors, and quads.

Why it's beneficial for you: Flexibility keeps your joints supple and expands your range of motion for daily tasks like playing with your grandchildren, tying your shoes, shampooing your hair, and checking behind you while you drive.

CHAPTER 2

You Can Build Muscle Strength At Any Age.

Muscle strength doesn't diminish as we age. Adults not only have the ability to combat the strength and muscle loss that comes with aging, but they may also use their golden years to build strength.

It is typical that your approach to exercise may change from when you were younger as your body ages. Instead of the other way around, our fitness routines should change as our bodies do. The same logic holds true for muscle development. In order to increase muscle mass as an older adult, one must modify exercise routines with the body in mind rather than spending hours lifting weights. This enables older persons to benefit from developing muscle mass.

The Importance of Building Muscle

We begin to lose roughly 15% of our lean muscle mass in our 30s. Our muscles support healthy aging and help us maintain overall well-being. For older persons, there are three main advantages to muscle growth:

Improves balance to reduce risks of falling

Reduces symptoms of aging problems, like osteoporosis

Lessens aches and pain from arthritis

Growing older increases your risk of falling and suffering an injury, thus having more muscle mass may reduce your risk of falling. More bone density also aids in reducing symptoms from common aging-related conditions like osteoporosis. Strength exercise, even a modest bit of it to build muscle, can increase bone density, which improves overall balance and strength. Our bones get porous as we age, which makes them more brittle and fracture-prone, and this is called osteoporosis. Strengthening the muscles around the bones while maintaining their health and resiliency through weight training. Similar to how aerobic exercise prevents cartilage between your joints from wearing down, strength training keeps joints from becoming stiff or painful. Your risk of developing the signs and symptoms of arthritis, lower back pain, and other joint aches decreases the more active and mobile you are.

How to Build Muscle Mass

To get the most out of your fitness regimen, it's important to maintain a good balance of nutrition, activity, and rest. Exercise is an important contributor to muscle growth in older persons.

Nutrition

Healthy eating entails more than just avoiding junk food. It entails ensuring that you are consuming the nutrients that your body needs. If you're an older adult asking how to develop muscle mass, think about your food as well as your exercise routine. Maintain a high fiber consumption, keep an eye on your calcium and vitamin D intake, and concentrate on three key areas.

Proteins: Your body uses proteins to grow muscle mass, so between 15 and 20% of your calories per day should come from them.

Carbs: Your body uses carbohydrates to produce energy; if you don't consume enough of them, your body will resort to muscle for energy. Too few carbs can prevent you from gaining muscle mass, while too many can make you gain weight.

Water: The body needs to be hydrated in order to effectively absorb all the nutrients it receives from meals, and nothing compares to the advantages of plain good H2O.

Activity

To gain muscle mass, exercise is essential, but the kind of activity matters. The two best approaches for an older adult to develop muscle mass are cardio and strength training.

Everyone needs cardio, but especially people who lead more sedentary lifestyles. It is essential for both metabolism and general heart health. Additionally, it doesn't have to be particularly taxing. Something low-impact, like biking or strolling, can be sufficient for older individuals.

For older folks, strength exercise is the key to muscle growth. The best way to accomplish this is slowly and with minimal weight. Your muscles must work harder when performing slow actions with lighter weights. Without a set of weights, you may perform resistance exercises like push-ups and squats using only your body weight.

No matter how active you get, you need to be sure to respect your limits and talents. The expert personal trainers at Excellence In Fitness will work with you to help you understand how your body functions and what is and isn't safe for it since as you get older, it can be more difficult to determine which exercises you can do safely and which ones you cannot.

Rest

Your muscles will be stretched to their absolute maximum during exercise, therefore it's important to give them time to recover. Do not exercise the same muscle groups twice in a row. Give your body a day or two to rest in between sessions. Make sure you prioritize relaxation as well if you don't want to end up hurting yourself. Not merely the days following your workout are crucial for rest. Additionally, you must do it right away after working out. Any workout program should be followed by a brief cooling down period to allow your muscles to unwind and your heart rate to return to normal. Stretching is a wonderful technique to accomplish this because it lowers the likelihood of soreness following exercise. To go one step further, the Excellence In Recovery program offers assisted stretching so you may reap the advantages of flexibility and full-body stretching without worrying about harm or injury.

How Long Does It Take Older Adults to Build Muscle?

Results in terms of fitness will differ from person to person. While it may just take a few weeks for some, for others it may take months. How fit you were beforehand and the composition of your body both affect how quickly you'll see results. The easiest method to see progress in yourself is to have clear, defined goals that you can concentrate on achieving. The truth is that there is no such thing as being too old when it comes to your health and well-being, despite the belief of some older folks that they are not young enough to be able to reach these kinds of fitness goals. There's no reason you shouldn't experience the results you desire and deserve as long as you're committed to increasing muscle mass as an older adult and you take care to work within your body's limitations. You can find a workout routine that works best for you and more precisely define your fitness goals by working with a personal trainer.

Get expert assistance, such as a few sessions with a personal trainer, if you can afford it. "This is the most secure method to begin." Start by performing eight to twelve reps at a weight that causes the muscles to get fatigued by the final few reps. Increase the frequency of your workouts until you are performing two to four sets of each exercise every other day. People with joint problems, such as arthritis, "may need adaptations," like performing more or fewer repetitions with a lighter weight. Ask for some first advice at your gym if you don't have a trainer or aren't experienced with weight-resistance exercises.

Always pay attention to your body. " Your body will try to notify you that something is wrong if it hurts or doesn't feel right. That whole notion of no pain, no gain is false."

Remain hydrated. Before and after exercise, drink water. Seniors should pay extra attention to this, according to Ms. Oestreich, who has observed that her older clients prefer to drink less water in an effort to reduce the number of trips to the restroom.

Eat sensibly. "You cannot out-exercise a lousy diet. While most people require about.8 grams of protein per kilo of body weight each day, those who have experienced a loss of muscle mass (known as sarcopenia) may require as much as 1.2 grams of protein per kilo of body weight. Eating protein before and after a workout will result in a better outcome for muscle growth and development. Here, you may convert your body weight from pounds to kilograms. (For example, a person weighing 165 pounds, or 75 kilos, needs at least 60 grams of protein per day, or up to 90 grams.)

Put on appropriate attire. "Footwear is especially crucial—sturdy sneakers with high traction and lace-up laces." Select breathable, loose-fitting shirts and shorts or pants.

Exercise as a group. "Working out in a group is a great opportunity to meet new people and get a great workout in a safe setting." It offers seniors social interaction at a stage in life when loneliness can be an issue. The human spirit benefits greatly from social interaction, according to this statement.

CHAPTER 3

Benefits of Exercise for Older Adults

We tend to slow down and become more sedentary as we age for a variety of reasons. It could be brought on by health issues, troubles with weight or pain, or concerns about falling. Or perhaps you believe that working out is simply not for you. But as you age, leading an active lifestyle is more crucial to your health than ever.

Physical exercise, according to a recent Swedish study, is the main factor in longevity, extending your life even if you don't start working out until you're in your senior years. However, being active will also give you more years to live, not just more years.

Moving around can help you feel more energized, keep your independence, preserve your heart, and control your weight as well as any disease or pain you may be experiencing. Additionally beneficial to your mind, mood, and memory is regular exercise. It's never too late to find easy, fun methods to increase your activity level, boost your mood and outlook, and benefit from all of exercise's positive effects on both your physical and mental health.

What are the benefits of exercise for older adults?

You've heard it time and time again: exercise and physical activity are healthy for you, and you should try to include them in your daily routine. Numerous studies have demonstrated the significant health benefits of exercise, which are amplified as we age.

Physical health benefits of exercise for seniors

As an older adult, exercise can help you to:

Maintain or lose weight. As you get older, your metabolism naturally slows down, making it harder to stay at a healthy weight. Regular exercise helps your metabolism rise and your muscles grow, which increases the number of calories your body burns.

lessen the effects of chronic illness and disease. Exercisers typically function better in the immune and digestive systems, have better blood pressure and bone density, and have a lower risk of developing conditions including Alzheimer's disease, diabetes, obesity, heart disease, osteoporosis, and some malignancies.

Improve your balance, flexibility, and mobility. Your balance and coordination will improve as a result of improved strength, flexibility, and posture, which can also lower your chance of falling. Strength training can also aid in reducing the signs and symptoms of long-term illnesses like arthritis.

Mental health benefits

Exercise can also help you to:

Improve your sleeping habits. As you age, getting enough sleep is crucial for your general health. Your ability to fall asleep more quickly, sleep deeper and wake up more energized and rested can all be improved with regular exercise.

Boost your disposition and self-esteem. Exercise is a great way to decrease stress, and the endorphins it produces have been shown to lessen depressive, anxious, and melancholy feelings. You can feel more confident by being active and feeling strong.

Boost your mental acuity Crossword puzzles and Sudoku can keep your brain engaged, but nothing compares to the advantages of exercise for the brain. It can help with memory loss, dementia, and a variety of other brain functions, including creativity and multitasking. Getting active may even help slow the progression of brain disorders such as Alzheimer's disease.

Regular exercise improves brain function

The discovery that the mind and body are much more interconnected than we would like to believe is one of the most amazing achievements in health science. According to a NCBI study, regular exercise among seniors has been linked to increased cognitive health since a healthy body equals a healthy mind. Regular exercise has been shown to cut the risk of dementia or Alzheimer's disease by almost 50%, according to a study by the Alzheimer's Research and Prevention Foundation.

Regularity means more energy

One gets fatigued from inactivity. On the other hand, being active makes you feel more energized.

Any level of physical activity encourages the release of endorphins, vital neurotransmitters associated with pain relief, and a positive mood. Endorphins help you feel more alive and energized while battling stress hormones and promoting sound sleep. It imparts a sensation of general well-being. Additionally, it lowers the levels of stress hormones in the body like cortisol and adrenaline, which aids in relaxation.

Reasons Why Elderly People Need To Exercise

An effective exercise regimen is one of the best ways to combat many of the unpleasant effects of aging. Exercise is important for older people for a variety of reasons, but one that stands out is that it can stop or even reverse many of the physical aging processes.

Seniors should engage in regular physical activity and exercise to maintain their physical and mental health, which will help them age independently. Ten reasons why elderly people should exercise are listed below;

1. Improved Mental Health

Exercise has a virtually limitless list of advantages for mental health. Exercise releases endorphins, the "feel good" hormone that reduces stress and makes you feel content and joyful. In addition, exercise has been related to enhancing sleep, which is especially essential for older persons who typically suffer from insomnia and irregular sleep patterns.

2. It keeps you fit.

The same study indicated that exercise helps prevent the emergence of several illnesses related to aging, including Type 2 diabetes and obesity.

3. It makes you sleep better.

According to a University of Warwick study, getting regular exercise during the day can help you sleep better at night. If despair or worry are the sources of their sleeplessness, senior exercises can also help them sleep better.

4. It keeps your joints working smoothly.

As we age, our muscles and joints deteriorate. We must balance our troops if we want to keep them operating effectively. According to a Canadian study, exercise helps seniors maintain their independence and mobility so they can live in their homes for longer.

5. It helps your body lose weight and fat.

Adults with obesity who participated in weight-loss programs had better results when they added regular exercise to them than when they only dieted or exercise.

6. It lowers your risk of heart disease.

According to a Harvard Medical Center study, regular exercise can lower your risk of heart disease by up to 30%.

7. It helps relieve stress and depression.

Our brain releases endorphins when we work out. Then, these contribute to improving our mood. Many people also discover that if they focus on engaging in physical exercises, such as working out at the gym or taking a brisk stroll in the park, they are more able to let go of their unwelcome worries.

8. It helps people cope with pain.

According to a University of Bristol study, exercise is a more effective pain management technique than drugs, yoga, or meditation.

9. It helps to prevent osteoporosis. Exercise maintains calcium levels in the body and raises amounts of vitamin D, which strengthens bones. All of these are essential for delaying the onset of osteoporosis in later life.

10. Decreased Risks of Falls

Falls are more likely to occur in older persons, which could be terrible for preserving independence. Exercise increases balance and coordination while also enhancing strength and flexibility, lowering the chance of falls. Fall recovery times are substantially longer for seniors, so anything that can be done to prevent falls in the first place is essential.

CHAPTER 4

Exercises For Seniors

According to the U.S. Department of Health and Human Services, exercise is important for older adults (age 65+) because it makes it simpler to carry out activities of daily living (ADLs), such as eating, bathing, toileting, dressing, getting into or out of a bed or chair, and moving around the house or neighborhood (HHS). Older persons who are physically active are also less prone to falls, which can result in catastrophic injuries.

Exercise increases bone density and muscle strength, which is crucial for women because they lose bone density more quickly than males do after menopause. In the meantime, the advantages of exercise for the heart and lungs support general health and reduce some risks for certain diseases and chronic conditions.

Types of exercises for seniors

It's crucial to consult a doctor before beginning an exercise program to make sure you're healthy enough for it and to learn which exercises are best for your current fitness level.

The types of exercises for seniors include the following:

1. Water aerobics

Water aerobics has recently gained enormous popularity among people of all ages, but seniors in particular. For people with arthritis and other types of joint discomfort, exercising in the water is perfect since the buoyancy of the water reduces the strain on your joints. Water also provides natural resistance, thus strength training doesn't require the use of weights. Your strength, flexibility, and balance will all increase thanks to water aerobics workouts, which put no strain on your body.

Excellent senior water aerobics exercises include:

Aqua jogging

Flutter kicking

Leg lifts

Standing water push-ups

Arm curls

2. Chair Yoga

Chair yoga, like water aerobics, is a low-impact exercise that enhances muscle strength, mobility, balance, and flexibility—all essential elements of senior health. A more accessible style of yoga than more traditional ones, chair yoga puts less strain on the muscles, joints, and bones.

Additionally, chair yoga has been demonstrated to enhance older persons' mental health. Regular chair yoga practitioners report better sleep, fewer cases of depression, and an overall feeling of well-being.

Excellent senior chair yoga exercises include:

Overhead stretch

Seated cow stretch

Seated cat stretch

Seated mountain pose

Seated twist

3. Body weight workouts

For older people, losing muscle can be heartbreaking and incapacitating. A third of elderly people suffer from severe muscle loss, which can cause hormonal imbalances, a reduction in protein metabolism, and other issues. One of the best strategies to combat the consequences of muscular atrophy in older persons is through bodyweight exercises. The affordability of body weight exercises is one of their main advantages. The equipment needed for bodyweight exercises is minimal; for the majority of bodyweight exercises, workout attire and a mat to cushion impact with the floor are needed.

Excellent senior body weight exercises include:

Squats to chair

Step up

Bird dog

Lying hip bridges

Side-lying circles

4. Five Easy Bed Exercises For Elderly

When you're stiff and exhausted, it might be difficult to set aside some time and effort, but we must never lose sight of how important exercise is to a healthy way of life.

However, you can perform a few exercises in bed to maintain your body's flexibility without getting out of bed. Here are 5 activities geared specifically toward those over the age of 55:

1) Knee bend with knees turned into chest: Perform this exercise to elevate your breastbone. As you do this, squeeze both your arms behind your back. For six seconds, maintain this posture; then, let go. Repeat 3 or more times.

2) Shoulder roll: Raise, lower, and then roll your shoulders to the left and right. Repeat ten times.

3) Leg stretch: Lift one leg and hold it straight up in the air for 10 seconds to stretch the leg. Without letting your knee touch the mattress, slowly drop it back to the bed. Make sure you don't relax your legs throughout this workout because it can lead to muscle tension. With your other leg, follow the same procedure.

4) Stomach massage: Repeat the following five times while lying on your back with your arms at your sides: - Pull in your stomach muscles for three seconds, then let them go.

- Raise your left knee to your chest, rub your stomach for 2 seconds, then let go and unwind. Do the same with your right knee.

5) Shoulder roll and neck stretch - Tilt your head as far to the right as you can, staring up at the ceiling. Simply maintain this stance for five seconds, then release and switch to the left.

The fact that you may perform these bed exercises for seniors in the comfort of your own home is their best feature. It is nonetheless important to understand that these workouts must be performed correctly and only after consulting a healthcare professional.

6. Five Core Exercises for Elderly

Even if you're in your 60s, just a few minutes of exercise can work miracles. Your health can be greatly improved by working out every day. Here are the five simplest core exercises that older individuals can undertake without hurting their backs.

1. Plank pose: Holding this position stabilizes the body's midsection while strengthening the arm and leg muscles. Additionally, if your lower back begins to suffer while you are performing this exercise, bend one or both of your knees so that they are directly beneath you, not in front of you.

2. Leg lift: While lying on your back with your knees bent, lift one leg up to about three feet off the ground, lower it to the ground, and then repeat with

the other leg. If necessary, grasp onto a chair to ensure your safety.

3. Modified cycling pose: By swaying from side to side, this exercise helps to develop the abdominal muscles. If done regularly, it also helps to loosen up the hip joints and buttocks, which can reduce lower back pain.

4. Standing chest stretch: With your elbows bent at 90 degrees, face a wall and place your hands on the wall. Stretch your arms and torso up against the wall while putting one foot in front of the other. Keep your head level with the ground the entire time.

5. Shoulder shrugs: Stand up straight, relax your shoulders, and then pull them up toward your ears while letting them drop down (not down and forward). Hold for a few whiles, then let them calm down once more. 10 times in a row (3 sets). Precaution: Avoid performing these exercises if you have high blood pressure or aneurysms. Consult

your doctor right away if you get even the smallest hernia symptoms.

7. Five Back Exercises For The Elderly to Try

Back discomfort is a typical issue that older persons deal with. They find it challenging to walk around and perform activities they used to do when they were younger because of their back pain. Fortunately, we have compiled a list of 5 simple and secure back exercises for seniors who are suffering from back pain.

1. Back Extensions. On your stomach, put your hands behind your back. Lift yourself 5 inches off the ground with your arms and hold that position for 5 seconds. then get back on the ground. Lift for three sets of ten.

2. Cat and dog stretch. The lower back and spine benefit greatly from this stretch. On all fours, arch your back as high as you can without lifting it off

the ground, tucking your chin into your chest at the same time. Hold for five seconds, then release. As often as you can throughout the day, repeat this 3-5 times.

3. Lay on your back with your knees bent. Put both hands on your back, directing the fingers in the direction of your waist. When you inhale deeply, run your fingers along your spine and massage it downward for 5–10 seconds before returning to the beginning position with your exhale. 3-5 times a day, repeat this cycle.

4. Knee bends. This exercise is beneficial for the glutes and lower back. Put your hands behind your head while lying on your back. While keeping the same alignment in the body, bend the right knee up toward the chest and then straighten it again. twenty times each day.

5. Leg lifts. This workout is beneficial for the glutes and back. Lie on your back and lift both legs so that

the lower leg is parallel to the floor. After holding for two seconds, bring them back down. Perform this workout 3-5 times per day.

Aging need not be unattractive and unhealthy. We all have the ability to age healthily with the aid of regular exercise. According to a study, people who are active live longer, have more energy, keep their mobility, and experience improvements in their mental health.

You can keep your freedom and reduce falls by staying active. By engaging in a regular exercise routine, you may strengthen your leg muscles to bring more balance to your body and enhance your posture. Strength training and increased aerobic ability also lower your chance of falling and suffering a fall injury.

Exercises Seniors Should Avoid

Many widely used and popular exercises are not recommended for older people. Younger folks wanting to bulk up or lose weight quickly will benefit from these popular exercises, but older adults who have joint discomfort, atrophied muscles, posture concerns, or challenges with balance may find them to be unhealthy.

If you're over 60, it's usually best to stay away from the following exercises:

Squats with dumbbells or weights

Bench press

Leg press

Long-distance running

Abdominal crunches

Upright row

Deadlift

High-intensity interval training

Rock climbing

Power clean

.

CHAPTER 5

Walking For Good Health.

Try to walk as briskly as you can for at least 30 minutes most days of the week to get the health benefits. "Brisk" refers to the fact that you can still converse but cannot sing and may be slightly exhaling. Walking is a moderate activity that poses little risk to your health, but if you have a medical problem, check with your doctor before beginning any new fitness program.

Your general health can be enhanced or maintained by walking. Everyday exercise for just 30 minutes can strengthen bones, improve cardiovascular fitness, lower excess body fat, and build muscle strength and endurance. It can also decrease your risk of contracting diseases like heart disease, type 2 diabetes, osteoporosis, and some malignancies. Walking costs nothing and doesn't call for any specialized gear or prior experience, unlike some other types of exercise.

Walking is a low-impact exercise that requires no gear, can be done at any time of day and may be done at your own pace. Without having to be concerned about the risks connected to some more strenuous forms of exercise, you can go for a walk. Walking is a fantastic kind of exercise for those who are overweight, old, or haven't worked out in a while.

Walking isn't just for leisurely strolling by oneself around your neighborhood streets. You can use a variety of groups, locations, and techniques to make walking a fun and social aspect of your life.

Health benefits of walking

Older folks can benefit much from walking. It can help you live independently for a longer period of time and can significantly enhance your health and wellness.

Walking can:

• Build physical activity into your life

If walking for 30 minutes at a time is too onerous, break it up into manageable 10-minute sessions every three hours and work your way up to larger sessions. However, you will need to engage in physical exercise for more than 30 minutes each day if your objective is to reduce weight. You can still accomplish this by beginning the day with little bursts of activity and building them up as your fitness level increases. One of the most effective strategies to aid in weight loss and help you keep the weight off once you've lost it is to incorporate physical activity into your everyday lifestyle.

- Strengthen your muscles.
- Help keep your weight steady.
- Lower your risk of heart disease, stroke, colon cancer, and diabetes.
- Strengthen your bones, and prevent osteoporosis and osteoarthritis (regular walking could halve the number of people over 45 who fracture their hip).
- Help reduce blood pressure in some people with hypertension.
- Improve your balance and coordination, and decrease your likelihood of falling.
- Keep your joints flexible.
- Increase your confidence and mood, and help you feel better all round.
- Improve your energy levels and increase your stamina.
- Reduce anxiety or depression.
- Improve your social life – walking is a great way to get out and meet people or socialize with your friends.

One of the best markers of whether someone can live independently is their ability to walk unassisted. Regular exercise increases an older person's ability to walk independently and perform tasks around the house.

Here are some ideas for building walking into your daily routine:

Take the stairs rather than the elevator (for at least part of the way).

Walk to work or home after alighting from public transportation one stop earlier.

To the neighborhood stores, walk rather than drive.

Walk your dog (or the dog that lives next door).

Walking while wearing a pedometer

Your daily step count is tracked using a pedometer. It can be used to track your daily activity and compare it to previous days or advised quantities. You could be inspired to move more as a result. To reap the benefits of daily activity on your health, aim for 10,000 steps or more.

A manageable degree of vigor for walking

For the majority of people, walking takes longer than running does, but there isn't much of a difference in the quantity of energy expended. Set a daily walking goal and keep track of how long it takes you to complete it. You will be able to walk farther and exert more energy as your fitness level increases.

Although walking quickly burns more calories per hour than walking slowly does not imply you should exert yourself to the point of exhaustion. Pace yourself so that you can still speak, instead. By following this straightforward guideline, you can walk comfortably while staying within your desired heart rate, which improves your health.

As you are able to boost your fitness levels, keep up the intensity of your physical exercise because our bodies have a tendency to get acclimated to it.

You can make your walks more challenging by:

walking up hills

walking with hand weights

increasing your walking speed gradually by including some quick walking

increasing the distance you walk quickly before returning to a moderate walking pace

walking for longer.

Warming up and cooling down after walking

Walking slowly is the ideal warm-up exercise. Each walk should begin slowly to allow your muscles to warm up, and then quickly increase in speed. Stretch your leg muscles gently afterward, paying special attention to your calves and front and back thighs. Ideally, stretches should be held for 20 seconds or so. Stop stretching if you experience any pain.

Avoid bouncing or jerking since you could overstretch your muscles and create microscopic tears, which will make them stiff and sore.

It's recommended to wear less clothing when exercising. Overdressing can make you sweat more and raise your body temperature, which can make a walk uncomfortable or even irritate your skin. Additionally, a gradual cool-down will avoid injury and muscle stiffness.

CHAPTER 6

Getting Started Safely

One of the healthiest choices you can make as you age is to get more active, but it's crucial to do it safely.

Before beginning an exercise program, seek medical approval from your doctor, especially if you have a pre-existing disease. Inquire about any activities you ought to steer clear of.

Consider your health. Be mindful of how your persistent medical issues affect your exercise regimen. For instance, diabetics may need to modify their food plans and prescription schedules in order to include exercise in their schedules.

Be aware of your body. Never should exercising hurt or make you feel bad. Stop exercising immediately and call your doctor if you feel dizzy or short of breath, develop chest pain or pressure, break out in a cold sweat, or have pain. The best method to deal with injuries is to prevent them in the first place. Delay your routine if a joint is red, swollen, or sensitive to the touch. If you frequently feel pain or discomfort after working out, try working out less frequently but for longer periods of time.

Start out slowly and steadily increase. Build up your fitness program gradually if you haven't been active in a while. Try dividing your two daily workouts into ten-minute intervals. Try taking just one lesson every week instead. Start with simple chair exercises to gradually improve your fitness and confidence if you're worried about falling or have a persistent heart condition.

Warm up, cool down, and have water close at hand to avoid injury and discomfort.

Set up a regular exercise program and force yourself to stick to it for at least three or four weeks so that it becomes a habit. If you find hobbies you enjoy, this is much simpler.

Try practicing mindfulness. Instead of losing yourself in your workout, try to pay attention to how your body feels as you move, such as the rhythm of your breathing, how your feet land, or the way your muscles twitch. Using mindfulness techniques will help you feel better physically, relieve stress and anxiety more effectively, and help you avoid accidents and injuries more effectively.

Support activity levels with the right diet

Your energy, mood, and fitness can all be significantly impacted by both diet and exercise. Many older adults do not consume enough high-quality protein in their diets, despite the fact that research indicates they require more of it than younger adults to support overall health, maintain energy levels, and maintain lean muscle mass. An ideal protein intake for elderly people without diabetes or kidney disease is 0.5 grams per pound of body weight.

Instead of relying just on red meat, diversify your protein sources by consuming more fish, poultry, beans, and eggs.

Reduce your intake of processed carbs such as cookies, cakes, pizza, cakes, pastries, and chips in favor of high-quality protein.

Replace chips with nuts and seeds as a snack, a baked dessert with Greek yogurt, and pizza pieces with grilled chicken breast and beans.

Tips for staying motivated

When illness, injury, or weather-related changes disrupt your routine and make it seem like you've lost ground, it's simple to become dejected. But even when difficulties in life get in the way, there are strategies to maintain motivation.

Goals like weight loss, which can take longer to attain, should not be your main focus. Instead, concentrate on short-term objectives like boosting your mood and energy levels and decreasing stress.

When you finish a workout, accomplish a new fitness goal, or simply show up on a day when you were tempted to cancel your exercise plans, treat yourself to something. Select something enjoyable activity that you save for after working out, such as a hot bath or a cup of your preferred coffee.

Keep a diary. Keeping track of your progress with a journal or an app not only keeps you accountable but also serves as a helpful reminder of your successes.

Find assistance. When you exercise with a buddy or member of your family, you can support and motivate one another.

Conclusion

Making exercise a priority and habit in your everyday life will help you reap the health benefits of exercise. Exercise has been demonstrated to increase mental health and well-being, reduce the incidence of falls, prevent disease, strengthen social bonds, and enhance cognitive performance in the aging population. Regardless of your age, we hope that this will encourage you to make fitness a part of your daily routine.